ABORTION RIGHTS MOVEMENT

Dr. Emmanuel Patrick

Dedication

To all women who are not aware of not aware
of their right towards abortion.

Table of Contents

Introduction

Abortion rights movement is a book that teaches women and educate them on the history and overview of abortion rights movement. It gives insight to women on their right as individuals towards abortion and preview of constitution laid down due to abortion.

A series of ongoing protests in support of abortion rights and anti-abortion opposition protests took place in the United States on May 2, 2022 after the leaked majority draft of the U.S.

Supreme Court's Dobbs v. Jackson Women's Health Agency case. It started with Roe v. Wade, thereby stating that the United States Constitution does not give the right to abortion.

 Wade and Planned Parenthood v. Casey. [1][2][3] On June 24, 2022, the Supreme Court officially overthrew Law and Casey at Dobbs, prompting further protests outside the United States Supreme Court building.

  The American Abortion Rights Movement (also known as the Pro-Choice Movement) is a socio-political movement in the United States that advocates the view that women should have a legal right to voluntary abortion.

terminate her pregnancy. and part of the broader global abortion rights movement. The movement is made up of various organizations that do not have a single centralized decision-making body. [1]

 An important point regarding the right to abortion in the United States was the 1973 decision of the US Supreme Court in the Roe v. Wade case. Wade invalidated most state laws that limit abortion [2] [3], thereby denying and legalizing voluntary abortion in many states. June 24, 2022, Roe v. Wade case. Dobbs v. Jackson's Wade Jackson

Women's Health Organization has been suspended.

 On the other side of the abortion controversy in the United States is the anti-abortion movement (which calls itself the "pro-life" movement). It believes that human embryos and fetuses have a right to life and that abortion violates abortion. It is law and must be prohibited or otherwise restricted. Within this group, many argue that human character begins at conception. This is a position opposed by many abortion rights groups.

Overview

Abortion rights advocates argue that whether or not a pregnant woman pursues a pregnancy should be her personal choice, as it concerns her body, personal health, and future. They also argue that the availability of legal abortion methods reduces a woman's risk for the risks associated with illegal abortion. More generally, abortion rights advocates frame their arguments about individual liberties, reproductive rights, and reproductive rights. The first of these terms was widely used to describe many political movements of the 19th and 20th centuries (such as in the abolition of slavery in Europe and the United States, and in the transmission of democratization of the people) while the following terms are derived from changing attitudes about sexual freedom and bodily integrity.

Abortion rights advocates rarely refer to themselves as "pro-abortion", because they see termination of pregnancy as a matter of physical autonomy, and consider forced abortion to be impossible. legal and ethical resistance such as banning abortion. Indeed, some abortion rights advocates consider themselves to be against some or all abortion on moral grounds, but believe that abortion happens anyway and that abortion is legal. under better controlled medical conditions than a clandestine illegal abortion without proper medical supervision. These people argue that the rate of women dying from such procedures in places where abortions are performed only outside of a medical facility is unacceptable.

 Some argue from a philosophical point of view that the embryo has no rights because it is only a potential person and not a real person and that it should not have any rights over the rights of a woman. get pregnant at least until it's feasible. .[4]

Many abortion rights activists also note that some anti-abortion activists also oppose activities related to lower demand for abortion, that is, sex education and availability willing to use contraception.

[5] [uncredited source] Supporters of this argument cite cases from areas with limited sex education and access to contraceptives and where abortion rates are high, for whether legal or illegal. Some women also go to other jurisdictions or countries for abortions.

For example, a large number of Irish women will go to the UK to have abortions, as will Belgian women to France before Belgium legalized abortion. Similarly, women traveled to the Netherlands when abortion became legal there in the 1970s. Situations where they believed abortion was a necessary option. These situations include cases where a woman has been raped, her (or unborn baby's) health or life is in jeopardy, contraception has been used without success, unborn baby has acute birth defects and disorders, incest, is in financial difficulty, or she feels incapable of raising a child. One of the most common reasons women give for an unwanted pregnancy is that having a baby will keep them from achieving goals like going to school.

[6] Some abortion-rights moderates, who would otherwise be willing to

accept certain restrictions on abortion, feel that political pragmatism compels them to oppose any such restrictions, as they could be used to form a slippery slope against all abortions.

[7][non-primary source needed] On the other hand, even some abortion rights advocates feel uncomfortable with the

use of abortion for sex-selection, as is practiced in some countries, such as India.

 The abortion rights movement includes a variety of organizations, with no single centralized decision-making body.[1]

Many more individuals who are not members of these organizations also support their views and arguments.

 Planned Parenthood, NARAL Pro-Choice America, the National Abortion Federation, the National Organization for Women, and the American Civil Liberties Union are the leading abortion-rights advocacy and lobbying groups in the United States. Most major feminist organizations also support abortion-rights positions, as do the American

Medical Association, the American Congress of Obstetricians and Gynecologists, and pro-abortion rights physicians such as Eugene Gu[22] and Warren Hern[23] who have fought political opposition from anti-abortion Senator Marsha Blackburn.[24][25] Faith-based groups that advocate for abortion rights include notably the Religious Coalition for Reproductive Choice and Catholics for Choice.

Planned Parent-Child Relationship

 Planned Parent-Child Relationship was established on October 16, 1916 in Brownsville, New York City, New York. This organization was established to give women access to medical services and information that help them lead a strong and healthy life.

 [26] Planned parent-child relationships are important to the US abortion movement. Because its members believe that abortion is a health care right, they support access to abortion. Some of the abortion-related issues that the organization opposes are 20-week abortion bans, 6-week abortion bans, and Hyde amendments.

July 1, 1976, Planned Parenthood v. Danforce in front of the US Supreme Court. Planned Filiation, Ph.D. in Central Missouri. David Hall and Dr. Michael Freiman challenged Missouri's abortion law, known as HouseBill1211, for minors and unmarried people. Attorney Frank Sussman represented the planned parent-child relationship in this case. [27] Hall, Freiman, Susman, and Planned Parenthood opposed HouseBill1211 and its definition of feasibility. They argued that there was a vague definition of viability that allowed the fetus to be considered viable, essentially making abortion illegal. It is also claimed that

House Bill 1211's passage is specifically targeted at individuals who wish to have an abortion by requiring the consent of their husband or parent for the abortion, rather than any other medical procedure.

[27]Other than Planned Parenthood's advocacy efforts for the abortion rights movement, their members also provide information at their clinics and website for the public. Regarding abortions, they make information available for those who may be considering abortions, information on the abortion pill, where

to find abortion clinics and what to expect when experiencing abortions.

NARAL Pro-Choice America

The NARAL Pro-Choice America Foundation campaigns against abortion, contraception, access to paid parental leave, and discrimination against pregnant women. [28] Its members provide education on the negative effects of policies against women's choices, support group policies, and advocate elections for high-ranking government officials to support those policies. Another division of the organization, the NARAL Pro-Choice America PAC, focuses on supporting political candidates who are willing to run for elections and defend their right to abortion. [28]

 The NARAL Pro-Choice America Foundation opposes targeted abortion laws (TRAPs), legal restrictions on access to abortions, and abortion denial laws. They were also part of a successful campaign to promote support for women's law and overall women's health. Includes Hellerstedt. Each women's law is a law created to abolish the Hyde amendment. This change will prevent women participating in government health programs such as Medicaid from receiving funding for abortion. The NARAL Pro-Choice Foundation has collected petition signatures in support of each women's law. [29] In the Supreme Court case, Whole Woman's Healthv. Hellerstedt of the NARAL Pro-Choice Foundation is campaigning for this proceeding. This particular case was brought to court because Texas regulations made it difficult for women to access abortion. The court ruled that this was unconstitutional. [30]

National Abortion Federation

The National Abortion Federation supports abortion providers in patient care. [31] Its members are committed to giving women choices regarding abortion, ensuring quality abortion care, and providing a platform for donors and patients to share their personal abortion experiences. increase. During the

COVID-19 pandemic, the National Abortion Federation campaigned to keep the abortion clinic open and considered it an essential service. The National Abortion Federation also provides a hotline to give patients access to abortion and financial support. They offer a patient partnership program that allows aborted people to share their personal experiences and stories with lawmakers. [32]

www.ingramcontent.com/pod-product-compliance
Lightning Source LLC
Chambersburg PA
CBHW080731120726
48001CB00010B/3195